The Health Benefits of Coconut Oil, Water & Jelly

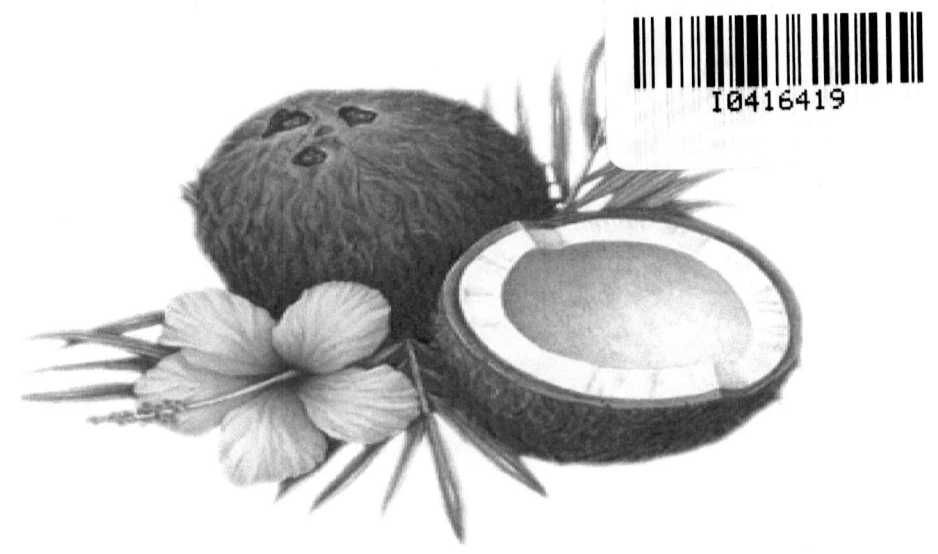

I0416419

Bishop Dr Juliette D. Fagan

Naturopathic Practitioner / Consultant

Cert. Clinical Colon Therapist

Copy Rights

ISBN 978-1-312-08314-1

Contents

The Health Benefits of Coconut Oil, Water & Jelly 1

Copy Rights 2

Acknowledgement: 4

Typical Caribbean Coconut Tree 6

Coconut Milk Medley 7

Introduction – The Coconut Myth 8

Chapter 1 – Coconut Oil and Your Hair 10

Pure Coconut Oil 11

Chapter 2 - Coconut Oil and Skincare 13

The Human Skin 15

Chapter 3 - Coconut Oil and Weight Loss 16

Raw Coconut in Husk 18

Chapter 4 – Coconut Oil as an Aid to Digestion 19

Chapter 5 – Coconut Oil as an Aid to the Immune System 21

Chapter 6 - Can Coconut Oil Help Fight Infections 23

Chapter 7 – Coconut Oil and Heart Disease 27

The Human Heart 29

Chapter 8 - Human Heart and Blood Pressure 30

Coconut Oil's Fantastic Natural Health Benefits 32

Coconut Milk 33

Caribbean Style Fat- Free Coconut Cake Recipe 34

New Book Release 35

About The Author 37

Special Thanks 39

Inspirational 40

Reviews 41

Speaking Engagements 42

Acknowledgement:

I want to give all honour and glory to Almighty God for bestowing His blessings and divine favor upon me over the years in so many ways. Special thanks to my darling husband Leeroy Fagan, a great support, partner, best friend, #1 chef and raw juice maker. Also to our children Jilliane Yunker, Julita Fagan, Leeron Fagan, relatives and our son in-law Daniel Yunker one Carib-Canadian who must have his coconut oil in the kitchen always. Thank you to all of the Bishops, Pastors and fellow brethren in the Lord Jesus Christ!

I just have to mention our two precious grandchildren, Trivon Scott and Malachi Yunker. Deaconess A. Powell (Sis Nicky) thanks for encouraging me to do this book and hanging in there during the good and bad times, Exhorter Bridgette Heron you have always been there to assist me technically over the years...Thanks! To all of you wonderful, praying, supportive and caring members at Vision Miracle Church of God, my family, friends and well-wishers all over, God bless you. Cathy Shae thanks for teaching and starting me off in the field of colon hydrotherapy as you can see it paid off. Woodrow Smallwood you are one of a kind, always encouraging and injecting new business ideas.

Amy Sanders you taught me so well at your clinical ColoLavage classes, thanks for choosing me as one of your ambassador for GPACT. Beth Seemann you are more than a friend, you are my sister in deed. Dr Christopher Demetriou

MD, Gastroenterologist, thank you and the GI Doctors team for training and certifying me in NYC, you really pushed me to the next level in the craft and the ability to be recognized and approved by the various health authorities.

Special thanks to the Cayman Islands Government Medical Council Board for approving me to practice as a Naturopathic Practitioner and Colon Therapist and The Ministry of Healthy Dept. Jamaica for approving Healthy Solutions as a natural health facility and colon therapy centre. Colon therapy is in the process of being regulated in these countries.

Last but not the least, Scooter Carter thanks for always checking in to see how I am doing over the years, always so encouraging, after all that's what friends are for. Bishop Lyndon Hutcherson, thank you sir, you really motivated me.

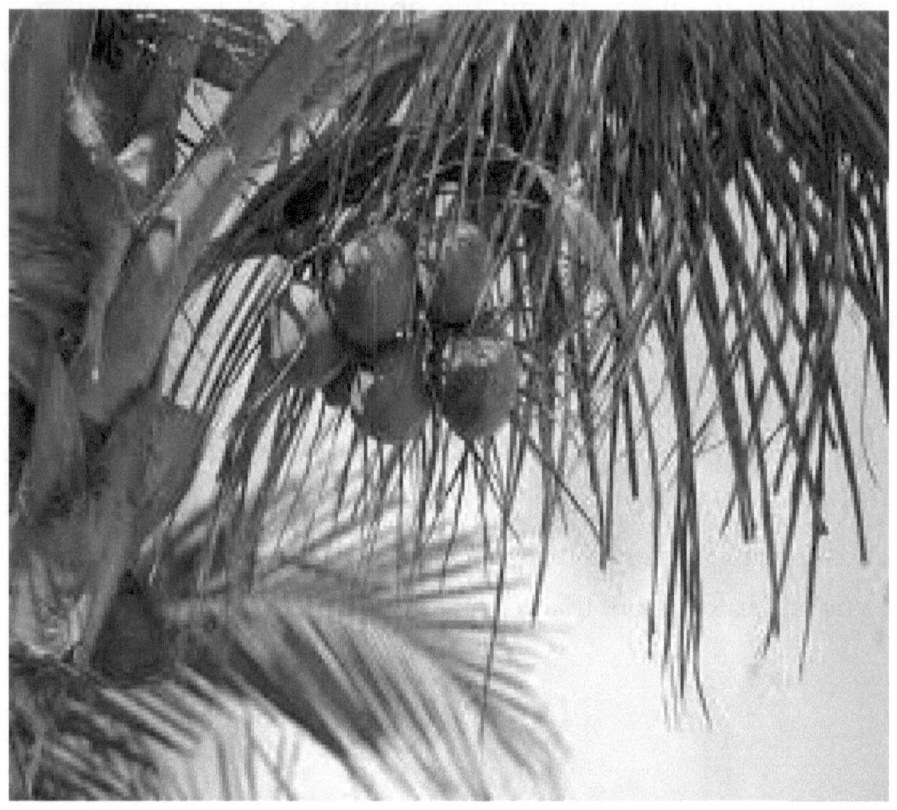

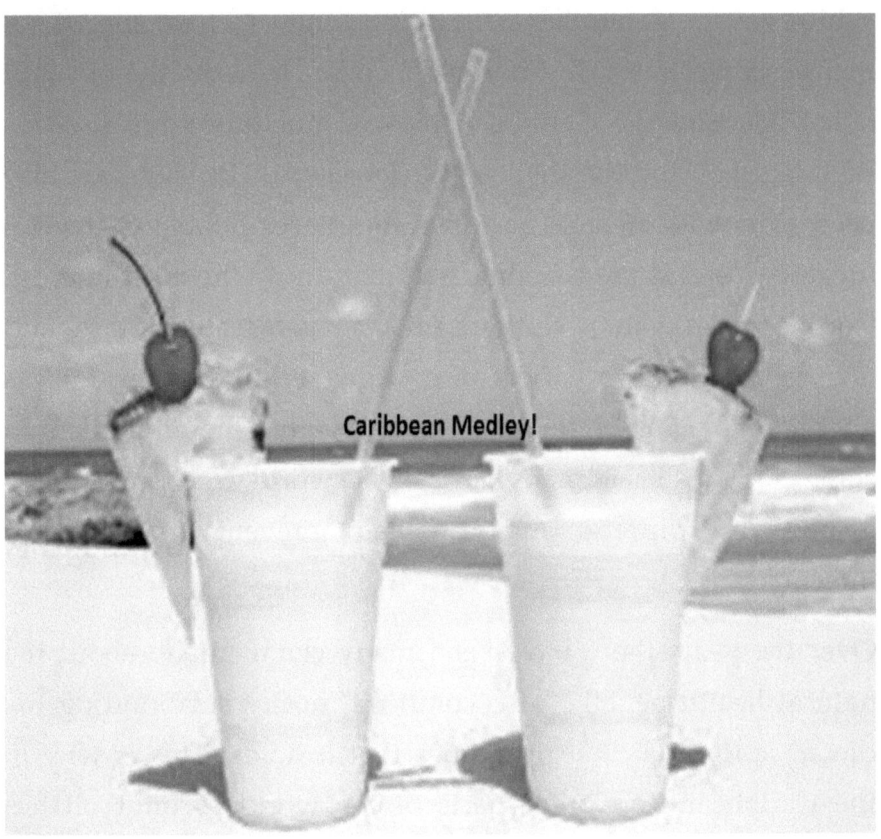

Caribbean Medley!

The coconut tree is one of the most versatile plants in existence. Whilst we are all familiar with the coconut as a food source not many people know the myriad of other benefits the coconut holds. Here in the Caribbean the coconut husks are used as floor brushes and the shell as fine jewellery. The shells are also used as bowls, utensils and in some places floatation devices for rafts. Yet it is the coconut itself that draws the most interest. Coconut flesh (jelly is soft and milky) has a beautiful taste and is used all over in a variety of cooking styles. Coconut milk is gorgeous to drink on its own and also is the chief ingredient in some curry dishes in many parts of the world. Coconut water is a powerful diuretic and can help prevent urinary tract infections.

Over the years there have been many claims made about the natural health benefits of coconut oil mostly surrounding the dietary and medicinal properties that it holds. This is why in the Caribbean and other parts of the world coconut oil has quickly become a hot consumer product with thousands of companies including it in their beauty products and thousands of recipes including it as an alternative to other oils.

Yet a lot of controversy still surrounds the actual health benefits of coconut and debates still exist as to whether claims of its benefits have been exaggerated. This is where this book comes into play. Over the years I have carefully researched the benefits of coconut oil and outlined at length all the fantastic qualities that can come from eating coconut, drinking the water, its cooking oil and applying it to your skin.

I have chosen to leave out some purported benefits due to lack of sufficient evidence to support them and hope that this book will go some way to dispelling the myths surrounding the health benefits of the coconut, whilst providing the reader with knowledge of coconut oil treatments that will be applicable to everyone in their normal lives.

Thank you for purchasing this book and Leeroy and I hope it will help you as it has and is still helping us. I will be focusing mainly on the coconut oil for now since that is a hot topic these days.

Coconut oil has long been regarded as one of the best hair conditioning natural health products in the natural world Many people worldwide use coconut oil as their sole hair conditioning product as it is relatively cheap and gives remarkable results.

The benefits of coconut oil for your hair are numerous. Coconut oil helps keep your hair fully moisturised, it promotes full growth and creates strong hair whilst keeping the scalp free from flakes. Its main benefit comes from increasing the protein retention in your hair – allowing for fuller and stronger growth. Coconut oil hot treatments are excellent for breaking, brittle hair.

Whilst many companies use tiny amounts of virgin coconut oil in their high end products a lot of people are now turning to pure virgin organic coconut oil for the benefits it brings. Stay away from additives as much as possible.

The key benefits of using coconut oil or even coconut oil cream in your hair can be exposed by looking at the chemical properties of coconut oil. As a trained Dudley's Cosmetologist, I often used and prescribed coconut oil as a remedy for hair loss when I operated my damaged hair clinic. I can testify that it slowed the onset of hairless areas and we will soon see why.

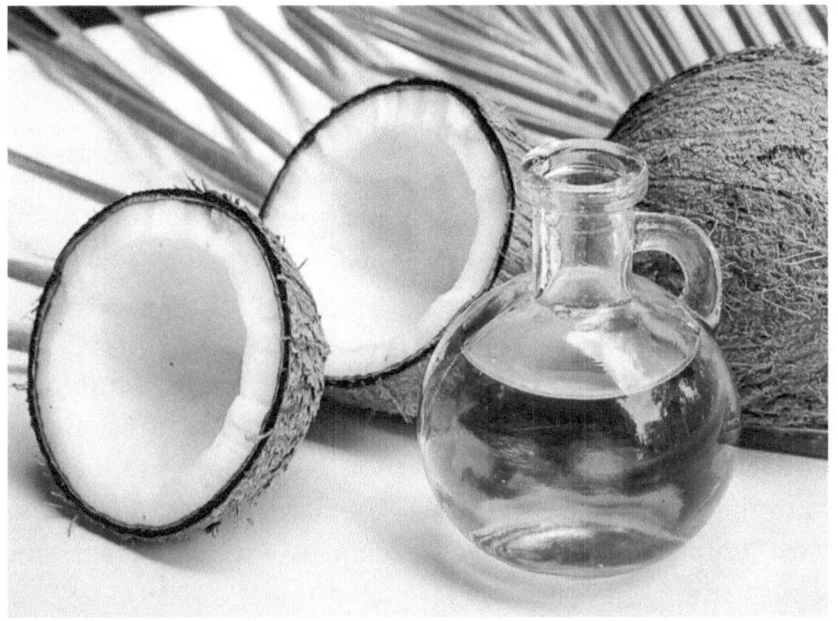

Lauric acid

Lauric acid is found primarily in the oil produced from coconuts. One of the primary causes of hair loss and recession of the hair line is the action of microbes on the scalp and at the base of the follicles. Lauric also acid acts as a antimicrobial oil that prevents the build-up of damaging microbes, thus preventing hair loss and stimulating fresh strong growth. This means that not only is coconut oil great for your hair but it can also prevent the loss of hair if used regularly as a scalp conditioner.

Capric acid

Virgin coconut oil contains a high yield of not only Lauric acid but Capric acid as well. Capric acid is another anti-microbe that works in a similar way to Lauric acid. It tackles microbes at the source preventing further spread and loss of hair whilst stimulating new hair growth.

Vitamin E

We all know how important vitamin E is to natural health generally. Vitamin E helps keep the skin in tip top condition and is one of the key ways in which your hair retains its shine and bounce.

Fatty acids

The fatty acids in coconut oil serve as a great anti-dandruff mechanism that far outshines most anti-dandruff shampoos. Regular application softens and moistens the skin reducing the accumulation of hair and flakes. The benefits of virgin coconut oil for your hair are fantastic. This is why more and more people are replacing their traditional shampoos and conditioners with either pure or high density coconut oil products. Many people have now started using coconut oil for stylistic reasons as it acts in a similar way to hair wax or gel without producing the flakes of typical wax and without damaging the hairs strength. This is due to coconut oils ability to retain moisture at almost all temperatures. Coconut oil also carries a natural and long lasting sheen.

Coconut oils natural health benefits extend far beyond the fantastic benefits for your hair that we just read about. Coconut oil has a large number of fantastic benefits for your skin as well.

The first as we have already seen is the great benefit of Vitamin E. Vitamin. Vitamin E keeps your skin healthy, spot free and protects against skin cancer.

Vitamin E found in coconut oil acts as an antioxidant - meaning that it protects skin cells from UV light, pollution and the negative effects of smoke and other "free radicals". The most notable of these is of course the prevention of skin cancer making coconut oil one of the most beneficial forms of sun screen available.

Vitamin E also helps reduce the appearance of stretch marks and prevents the appearance of age spots by rejuvenating the skin cells over your body.

As coconut oil has a high yield of vitamin E many people are now using it as a substantive replacement for expensive sun-creams, or as a supplement to sun screen as it is less harmful to the skin and has a pleasant scent.

Coconut oil also has fantastic moisturising benefits that extend beyond simply the high content of vitamin E.

Virgin coconut oil is a highly effective and completely natural moisturiser. It is unlikely to create adverse reactions as it is completely natural meaning that, unlike many moisturisers, you don't have to worry about allergies, rashes and unsightly blemishes appearing on your skin. Further compared to most moisturising creams - which let's face it carry extortionate price tag – coconut oil can be made at home and is cheap to buy and lasts a long time.

In terms of natural remedies coconut oil treats and alleviates many common skin conditions including eczema, dermatitis and psoriasis. This is why it is common ingredient in skin treatments worldwide. So by now you are probably thinking this is great I'll buy some, but there's actually more benefits to your skin from coconut oil still to come.

Finally, on the skin coconut oil actually works as an anti-ageing cream. The antioxidants of vitamin E provide an initial layer of protection against the sun but the combination of this with the Lauric acid found in coconut oil keeps the skin bacteria free. This means that coconut oil is giving your skin a double helping of beneficial effects. This promotes anti-ageing skin as it fights off bacteria and strengthens the skin tissue. Not the same on bleached skin.

Coconut oil really is a one of nature's most wonderful products and in the next chapter we'll see more.

The Skin Layers

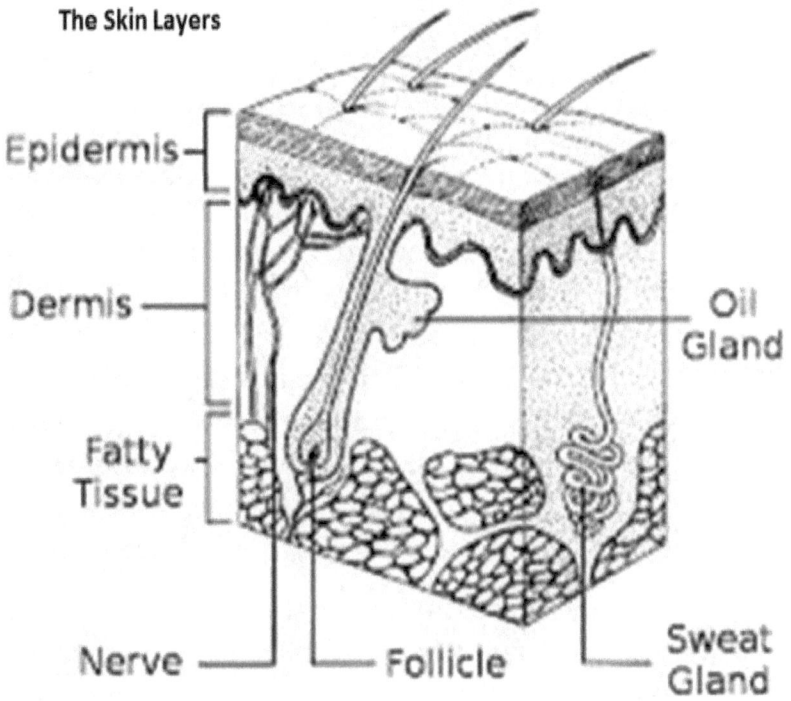

Many people think that because virgin coconut oil has a high proportion of saturated fat it is bad for you to eat. This is one of the greatest myths surrounding coconut oil and after much research and use myself I now turn to dispelling this myth and seeing how you can use coconut oil as a an aid to weight loss and other health benefits.

The chemical make-up of coconut oil is 90% saturated fat. Processed cooking oils are where the health danger lies. I know the word saturated fats sounds like a nightmare, doesn't it, but a closer examination reveals the surprising truth. This is because most of the saturated fatty acids in coconut oil are what is known as medium chain triglycerides. Medium chain triglycerides are actually easier for your body to break down and readily absorb than other saturated fats, especially those found in fast food and other artificially created products.

This is because there are fundamental differences in the chain composition in these fats which mean they are harder for your body to breakdown - which in turn means they are more likely to accumulate in your arteries and in your skin tissue as adipose tissue or excess fat.

Furthermore, the saturated fats in coconut oil - especially the Lauric acid actually increase the body's metabolism and promote optimal health of the thyroid and enzymes systems. Having a high metabolism means that the body burns calories at an increased rate. This is due to the acidity of your stomach acid and how effectively it can convert food to energy. Having a healthy gut (colon) will greatly increase your chances of having a high metabolism and help you start shedding pounds and losing weight. That's why I recommend a series of colonics for all of my clients before going on any kind of weight loss program and for overall health benefits. An improperly functional and impacted colon impedes the entire body, organs and systems.

Do you suffer from burning stomach? I have good news. The enzymes contained within coconut oil actually act as catalysts to your stomach acid and help you break down fat at an increased rate - and as your metabolism is also increased you can burn a higher proportion of the calories you take in. They also help to promote a healthy gut by fighting bacteria and strengthening the stomach lining. Hence coconut oil actually is much better for you to use in cooking and food than other alternatives as it has added benefits not found in vegetable and olive oil. Virgin coconut oil contains 50% lauric acid is definitely well worth including in your diet. The easiest way to do this is to replace your cooking oil with good ole, natural coconut oil like our fore parents did - which incidentally is much more complimentary to the tastes of many foods, especially rice and peas, curries, fish run down, stew peas, stir-fry's and several other dishes here in the Caribbean and world-wide. Alternatively you can also use coconut milk more regularly in your cooking as it can be a key ingredient in a variety of delicious dishes and for baking. Coconut oil is a must in mostly every home and restaurants in the Caribbean.

Virgin Coconut Oil, Lemon Juice, natural seasoning and spices can be made into a great tasting salad dressing.

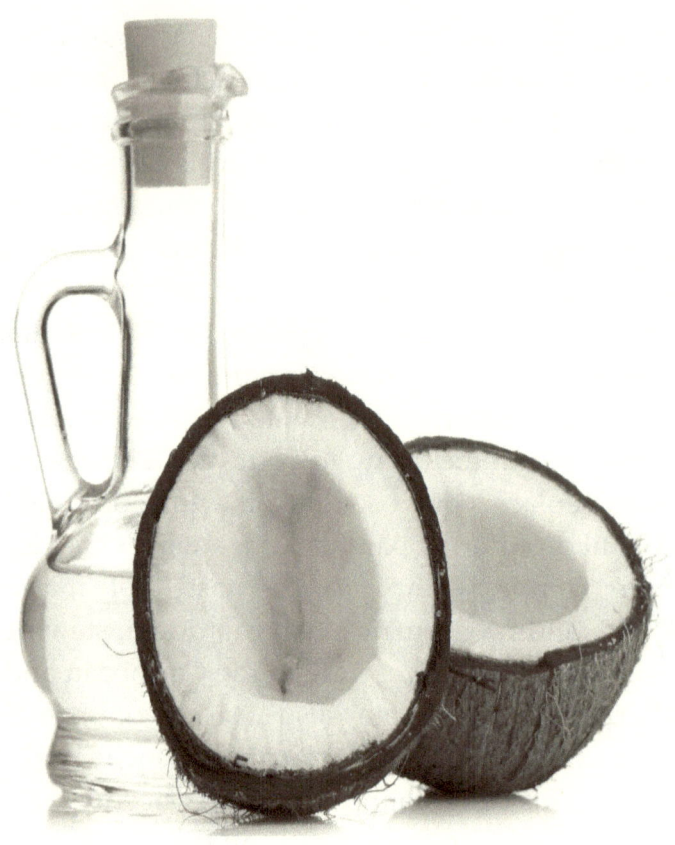

Coconut oil has long been held to be a useful supplement to aid in digestion. This is one of the key reasons it is the primary ingredient in many curry products and why curry goes down and is digested so well.

As we have seen in previous chapters coconut oil has strong anti-microbial benefits which when ingested help you to fight off nasty bacteria and bolster your immune system. The immune system is constantly under attack and needs all the help it can get.

Many digestive problems are caused by the presence of microbes in the food we eat, and especially all of the "fast processed food" preparations. We have a natural set of microbes in our stomach acid that aid digestion but these often react negatively with certain enzymes found in other foods. This means that the key way virgin coconut oil can help our digestion is by preventing and curing indigestion.

Indigestion is primarily caused by acid in your stomach irritating the stomach lining and the top of your small intestine. The most common process that causes it is known as acid reflux (burning stomach). This is most commonly caused by bad diet, obesity, poor colon health due to constipation as well as stomach ulcers and other stomach infections.

The saturated fats in coconut oil, especially Lauric acid and Capric acid, aid your stomach, and digestive track, in neutralising micro bacteria. These fats help remove parasitic bacteria and fungi keeping your digestive track, stomach and colon at its optimal performance. Whilst these benefits are great if you have indigestion they also help the clean and healthy running of the rest of your body too. Virgin, natural coconut oil is rich in vitamins and minerals itself but the fatty acids within it actually encourage the absorption of most other vitamins and minerals into your body enzymes that are released when the fatty acid chains break down act as a catalyst for the absorption of other vitamins and minerals.

<u>Caution</u>: Before you go guzzling gallons of coconut oil be aware that this could have a negative impact on your overall health. Whilst coconut oil is a great way to cure indigestion and is beneficial to your digestive system in general, over-use of coconut oil can have negative consequences. This is because whilst the saturated fats in virgin coconut oil are not unhealthy in small doses large amounts will be equivalent to eating lots of unhealthy meat and dairy products. So it is best to use coconut oil in cooking without pouring the entire bottle over every meal. Moderation in all things is the key to success.

Maintaining a well-balanced diet and carefully monitoring your daily food and drink intake are central to keeping a well-balanced and healthy immune system. Your immune system has to fight off scores of bacteria every day and having a low immune system means you are more likely to catch viruses and other illnesses.

Ingesting coconut oil, drinking coconut water and eat it can help your immune system in a surprising number of ways. As we've already discussed coconut oil has great natural health benefits and works as an effective cure for a number of common illnesses including eczema, indigestion, colon health and a variety of skin diseases like age spot. However coconut oil can also aid your immune system in a number of surprising ways.

The key way coconut oil can boost your immune system is through the ingestion of saturated fats - the most beneficial of which are - medium chain triglycerides. These are the most easily digestible saturated fats as the body transports them straight to the liver where they are not used for the production of fat, so you don't have to be overly worried about increasing your cholesterol as you boost your immune system. HDL or "high density lipoprotein" or "good cholesterol" and LDL or low density lipoprotein is called the "bad cholesterol" because it does not aid in transporting cholesterol out of the body, but instead deposits cholesterol onto the blood vessel wall which causes a narrowing and prevention of proper blood flow.

Medium chain triglycerides are used by your immune system to create antimicrobials - which we more commonly think of as antibodies. Antibodies are the primary defence mechanism your body has when fighting infections due to bacteria, fungus and viruses. Having moderate amounts of saturated fats is necessary to keep your antibody production up.

The fats in coconut oil contain antimicrobial lipids which have anti-viral and anti-fungal properties. Coconut oil contains Lauric, Caprylic and Capric acids which, when broken down, are converted into specific antibodies used to in your body's defences against a range of diseases including herpes, influenza and other infections / diseases. Having the right antibodies to fight specific bacteria is central to your body's wellbeing so adding some coconut oil to your diet is an easy way to ensure you stay happy and healthy.

We've already seen that coconut oil can help fight a variety of infections and that it aids your immune system thanks to the fatty acids such as lauric acid and capric acid. However the natural health benefits of coconut oil actually go far far beyond this as it is a versatile treatment for a variety of internal and external infections. It is these we are going to examine in this chapter.

Firstly, externally coconut oil can be used to treat a variety of skin afflictions and is brilliant for cuts, scrapes and bruises. Bleaching your skin with carcinogenic chemicals destroys the two natural protective layers of the skin (epidermis and dermis) which cannot be replaced but requires serious protective measures from skin cancer and other toxic effects.

On your natural God given skin, virgin coconut oil is aptly suited to preventing common skin afflictions such as eczema, dryness and other rashes as it creates an impermeable layer of oil between your skin and the air. Whilst usually this would result in your skin becoming unhealthy and not being able to breathe properly the natural chemical composition of coconut oil actually aerates the skin, softens and moisturises it at the same time.

You shouldn't keep yourself covered in coconut oil twenty four seven but applying a layer twice a day will keep your skin irritations safely at bay and leave you with healthier beautiful and softer skin no matter what colour it is.

On cuts, bruises and scrapes virgin coconut oil helps in the same way as above by keeping the area free from infection. Yet the moisturising effects also help heal the skin by giving it the nutrients it needs to rejuvenate, repair and restore the skin tissue. The nutrients in coconut oil not only help heal your skin but they also help tighten the skin - this is great for removing stretch marks and minimising scar tissue.

Secondly, the enzymes in coconut oil are known to stop the effects and even kill many viruses including influenza, measles, herpes, hepatitis and many others. This means that coconut oil can actually protect you from catching some of the worst diseases we are exposed to in the modern world. The enzymes work by simply decomposing (breaking down) the harmful bacteria, there by neutralising any potential they have to create negative effects.

Thirdly, coconut oil is a great treatment for candidiasis and other yeast or fungal infections. Candida Albicans (yeast) is the most common cause of fungal infections especially in women. Candida is a form of yeast, and every human being has a small amount of yeast as it lives in our mouth and intestine (colon) Men also have yeast and can pass in on through semen during sexual intercourse.

When yeast is kept under control it actually aid with digestion and nutrient absorption. But, when there is an overgrowth, candida destroys the wall of the colon and penetrates into the blood stream, releasing toxic waste or by-products into your body and this is called leaky gut. Leaky gut can lead to leaky gut syndrome which in turn can lead to many different kinds of health problems in males and females. The best thing one can do to correct a leaky gut and get rid of chronic bouts of yeast infections is a series of colon hydrotherapy followed by a good strain of probiotics, and lower your sugar intake including some fresh fruits. I will be doing another book on the health benefits, cons and pros of colon hydrotherapy in the near future.

Fourthly, coconut oil in its natural organic form is the best vaginal lubricant for menopausal women who are prone to dryness and painful intercourse. To all of you couples out there. This is not what I read about recently but what I have been using personally for many years with good results. Leeroy has found a way to make his own lubricant and it works just fine.

Back to coconut oil, as I said before organic coconut oil is one of the most efficient natural health aids in fighting candida off completely. Colon cleansing and changing your diet in this simple way can really help relieve you of repeated candidiasis.

Candida is notoriously hard to remove from the body as the source of the infection is not necessarily the same as the location of the infection itself due to entering the bloodstream after permeating the colon wall. That's the reason women experience yeast infections repeatedly.

Candida grows in a low PH (acidic environment) and overly toxic environment. If you are overweight, eat a lot of junk food or underweight and sedentary your bodies skin and immune system are less tolerant, meaning you are likely to develop candida or yeast infections much more frequently. Antibiotics and most pharmaceutical drugs are acidic and only serve to destroy the remaining good gut flora and decrease the immune system. Nevertheless, I am speaking from a natural health practitioner and clinical colon therapist perspective.

In your diet coconut oil helps bolster the immune system as well as being a much better source of saturated fat than junk food helping you to actually lose weight whilst still maintaining a balanced diet. It also makes great salad dressing.

Review, applied externally the nutrients in coconut oil help to protect your skin and create a barrier to external free radicals meaning that repeat infections are unlikely. The topical application of coconut oil will also help soothe the skin meaning you won't suffer from as much irritation. Coconut oil acts as a fungicide by literally breaking down the fungus and halting further fungal growth. This makes coconut products one of the best natural health remedies to a huge variety of common afflictions. It really is a wonder of the natural world and you'd be remiss not to buy and start using, drinking and eating some today.

Chapter 7 – Coconut Oil and Heart Disease

In this last section we're going to be examining the claimed benefits of coconut oil in relation to the prevention of heart disease. This is perhaps the most widely contested area of debate in all of the coconut oil research. The high amount of saturated fats in coconut oil would seem to indicate that it would have a negative impact on your health by creating more fatty tissues. However research into the chemical composition of these saturated fats has shown that they are primarily medium chain triglycerides, the least harmful, and most beneficial, form of saturated fats your body can use.

Worldwide cardiovascular disease causes over 12.5 million deaths a year whilst in many first world countries over 60 million people suffer some form of cardiovascular (heart) disease. The most common form of this disease is coronary artery disease which results from the build-up of fat, plaque and scar tissue around the arteries due to bad fats or LDL cholesterol called Arteriosclerosis.

The most common causes of cardiovascular disease are;

* High cholesterol (bad cholesterol)

* Heredity (genetically passed on to child)

* Smoking (including second smoke)

* Obesity (overweight for age and height, eating disorder)

* High blood pressure (narrowing of arteries and other heart issues)

* Diabetes (poor functioning pancreas to produce enough insulin)

This means that coconut oil would seem an unlikely candidate as a dietary supplement to decrease your risk of heart disease but it actually isn't.

This all has to do with the type of saturated fats we ingest on a regular basis. I recently found out that in Sri Lanka which has the lowest risk of cardiovascular disease in the world, with their primary cooking oil coming from coconuts. This may seem incidental but there has been a marked increase also in cardiovascular disease in Sri Lanka and India that fits with the increased use of other on the market vegetable oils among the younger generation which have replaced traditional cooking oils and consumables for processed foods.

The saturated fats in most Caribbean and western diets are of a far worse kind. These are high chain triglycerides that the body cannot absorb or break down as efficiently as medium chains. This means that they build up as fatty deposits around your heart and arteries increasing the risk of coronary heart disease. Replacing your oils and margarines with natural coconut oil therefore actually decreases your risk of heart disease and will help you lose weight also.

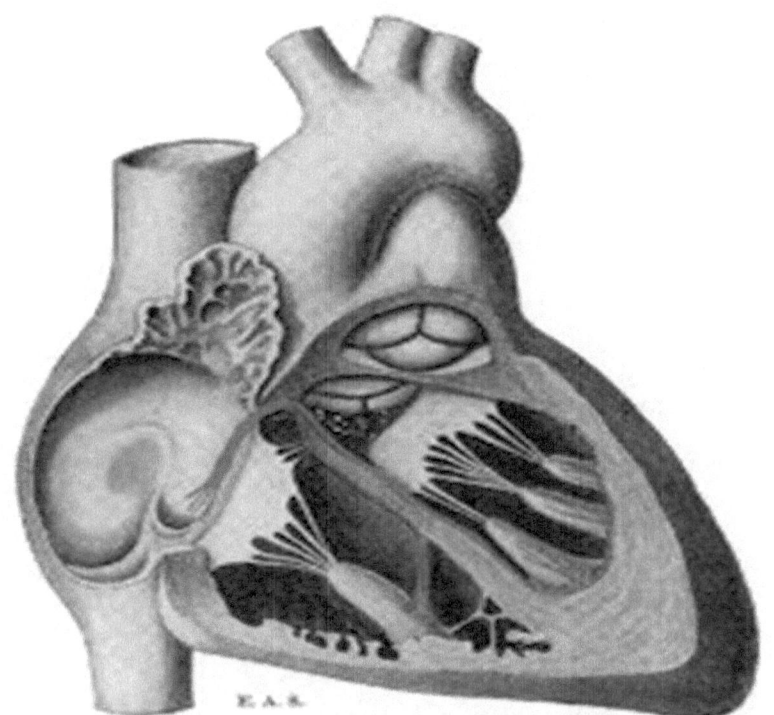

The Human Heart and blood flow

The human heart is a vital organ that acts as a pump; it provides a continuous flow of blood through the body. High blood pressure and arteriosclerosis (hardening of the artery walls due to fat build up) are the two most common heart diseases.

Blood Pressure Readings:

Hypotension - <90 / <60

Normal blood pressure – 120 / 80

Prehypertension – 139 / 89

Hypertension (stage1) – 140-159 / 90-99

Hypertension (stage2) 160-180 / 100-110

Hypertensive Crisis - >180 / >110 (Emergency Care Need)

In the event of narrowing or hardening of the arteries due to being plugged with fatty substances, the flow of blood is restricted and the heart does not get sufficient oxygen.

If the narrowed arteries get blocked due to a clot or thrombus inside them, causing death of that portion of the heart which depends upon the choked arteries, it is called a heart attack or coronary thrombosis. It may lead to death or heal, leaving a scar.

Clearly then we can see that despite all of the myths out there, the fact remains that coconut oil is a better choice. Coconut oil is actually a better alternative to other oils and should definitely be used as often as possible in order to improve your diet, digestion, skin, colon, hair, arteries, blood flow, reduce the risks of heart diseases and as I said as a natural lubricant.

Coconut water hydrates and is a great tasting alternative to sodas and energy drinks which are deadly. It is also a natural diuretic (increases urine) and is a great source of electrolyte such as potassium which helps with muscle contraction and generates energy.

Coconut water and jelly is very rich in nutrients like calcium, magnesium, phosphorus and natural sodium that the body readily needs for proper electrolyte functions. Like everything else do everything in moderation.

The Coconut and its oil, water and jelly is really one of nature's most wonderful products. It can help out in so many ways with your diet, health and overall hygiene that we should all be encouraged to switch and improve our overall well- being. Giving yourself a well-balanced diet, regular colon hydrotherapy, lots of water, probiotics, fibre, enzymes, rest, essential oils, exercise, positive attitude, prayer, fasting and doing the best you can for your body is central to living a long, healthy and fruitful life as God created you to do.

The fact that coconut oil can also treat a variety of common afflictions and illnesses serves only to strengthen the need to have some handy at all times.   I am not a university trained medical doctor. Contact and follow your medical doctor before starting any kind of dieting.

I hope you find this practical guide to the benefits of one of nature's gem "the good-ole coconut" useful for many years to come. Grow what you and eat what you grow. Henceforth, let natural organic foods be your medicine, exercise regularly, sleep well, drink lots of water, detoxify your body and maintain a healthy heart. Trust in the Lord, with all of your heart; and lean not on your own understanding. In all of your ways acknowledge Him, and He will direct your paths Proverbs 3:5-6.

Coconut Milk

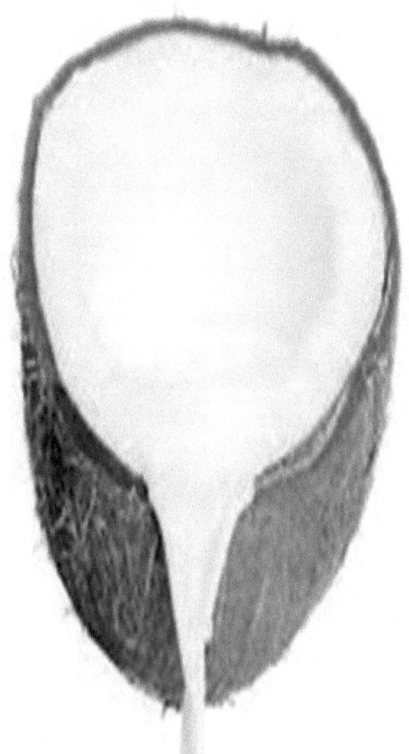

Fresh Coconut milk great for cooking, baking and drinks

Caribbean Style Fat- Free Coconut Cake Recipe

1 cup white flour

2 cups whole wheat flour

1 cup coconut oil

2 cups flaked coconut

1 teaspoon salt

2 cups brown sugar

2 teaspoons mixed spice

2 teaspoons baking powder

1 teaspoon baking soda

1 teaspoon vanilla

6 eggs

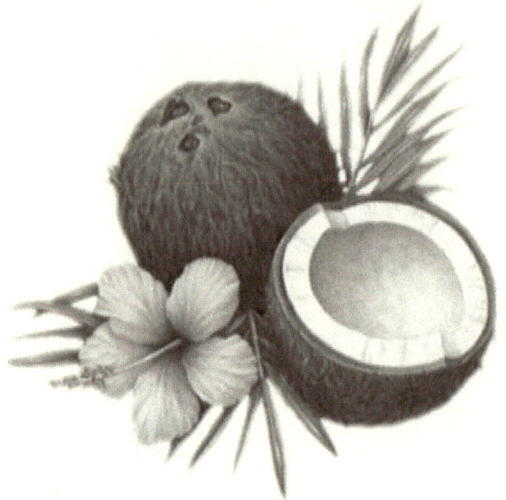

1. Sift all the dry ingredients together

2. In a blender whip the eggs, cooking oil and vanilla until creamy

3. Toss the flaked coconut into the dry ingredients until evenly spread

4. Add the liquid to the dry ingredients and mix until well combined

5. Pour into a greased and lined 9inch tin

6. Bake in a pre-heated 350 degree oven for about 45 to 60 minutes

7. Cool and serve

Contributed by: Pastor Jacqueline Chin-DePass, Caribbean International Chef of Jamaica.

Let Food Be You Medicine!

Relieving Irritable Bowel Syndrome Naturally!

Get these fantastic book today and find out why more and more people are switching to raw juice fast for weight lost, learn more about the alkaline diet, the cause of most irritable bowel syndrome disorder, the dangers of too much acid in the body and how to regain optimum health.

Would you like to know why it is that processed food is responsible for thousands of health problems all over the world?

Do you want a healthier diet?

Do you want to know exactly which juices have the best benefits for certain ailments and how to combine them?

Do you want to boost your immune system, so you can fight off illness and disease in a completely natural way?

It is a fact that raw food forms a substantive part of our diets wherever we are in the world. Yet knowing which fruit and vegetable to eat hold the greatest health benefits is not so easy.

Most people know that if you boil certain vegetables you will lose some of the vitamins and minerals they contain. But did you know that there are some vegetables that are actually better for you as raw juice, or marinated using certain oils.

After having the information, I decided to start writing my healthy life style books. Get your copy today!

Dr Juliette Fagan's Best Sellers

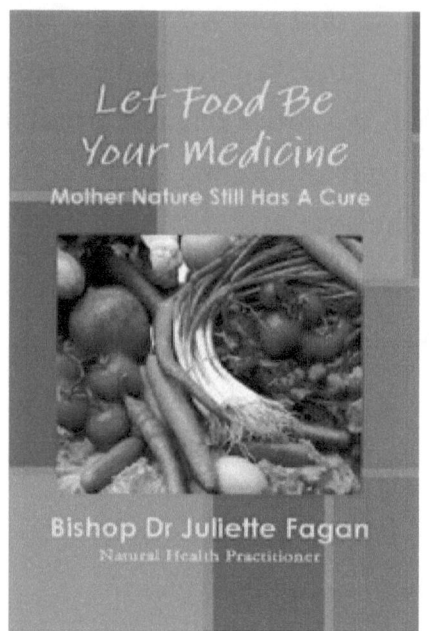

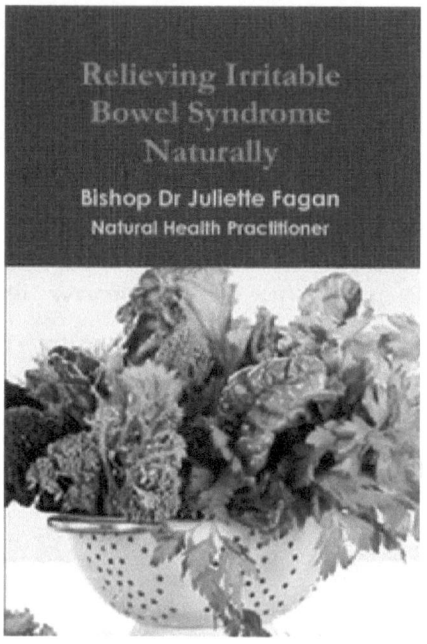

Bishop Dr. Juliette D. Fagan, Prof. Native born Caymanian, married to Pastor Leeroy Fagan. Owner and CEO of Healthy Solutions Colon Therapy and Detoxification Centres located in Jamaica and Grand Cayman. Dr Fagan as she is affectionately called is a trained Practical Nurse, Cayman Islands School of Nursing, and Ex-Police Officer with The Royal Cayman Islands Police Force. She is also a gospel recording artist with two albums. She became the first Caymanian woman pastor and first ordained Bishop in the Cayman Islands. She was A true pioneer for women in ministry in the Cayman Islands in the late 80's.

Studied Surgical Technology at Lindsey Hopkins Technical Miami Fla, Naturopathic Practitioner and Consultant at the Alternative Medicine of College of Canada, Colon Hydrotherapy, The International School for Colon Therapy USA, Clinical Colon Hydrotherapy, GI Doctors, Garden City NY with Amy Sanders of GPACT, Caribbean Ambassador of Global Professional Association for Colon Therapists. She is a certified Prepare & Enrichment Family and Marital Counsellor Fla, Marriage officer Cayman Islands Government.

Dr Fagan is the founder and President of Vision Miracle Church of God Evangelistic Association and Vision Dominion School of Theology. Graduate of the International Seminary USA, Professor of Theology, Christ Kingdom University Cameroon Africa. Radio and TV personality, author, inspirational, columnist and healthy life styles Speaker.

Married to Pastor Leeroy Fagan, have 3 children and 2 grandchildren.

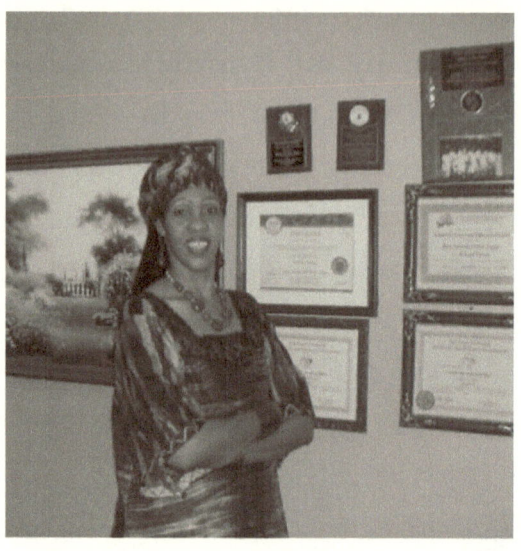

Bishop Dr Juliette D. Fagan, Prof. of Theology
Naturopathic Practitioner & Cert. Clinical Colon Therapist

Special Thanks

To everyone who constantly encouraged and inspired me to do this book after my articles, seminars, talk shows, consultations and testimonies about Leeroy's great cooking, baking and our belief in coconut oil, coconut water and jelly. I hope this small but compact book has been educational and enlightening to you.   Look out for more of my educational, inspiring and uplifting books. Last but not the least, Michael Gibbons thanks for assisting me on this project, your patience has paid off.

3 John 2

Behold, I wish above all things that you may prosper and be in health, even as your soul prospers. Make sure you always have coconut oil in your kitchen.

Isa 55: 9-11

9 for as the heavens are higher than the earth, so are my ways higher than your ways, and my thoughts than your thoughts. 10 For as the rain cometh down, and the snow from heaven, and returneth not thither, but watereth the earth, and maketh it bring forth and bud, that it may give seed to the sower, and bread to the eater: 11 So shall my word be that goeth forth out of my mouth: it shall not return unto me void, but it shall accomplish that which I please, and it shall prosper in the thing whereto I sent it.

1 John 5:14-15

"And this is the confidence that we have in him, that, if we ask any thing according to his will, he heareth us: And if we know that he hear us, whatsoever we ask, we know that we have the petitions that we desired of him.

Have a healthy, prosperous and blessed day!

Reviews

I encourage you to buy this book as I found it to be very informative and I learnt a lot from it. Scooter Carter, Virginia

As a school teacher and author myself I can say I am impressed with the amount of information that is packed in this small but powerful book. This is one book you need to have in your library collection. Althea Grizzle, Author, Educator. Jamaica

There is a time and season for everything and this is the time and season for the release of this awesome book on the health benefits of coconut oil. I am so excited to see one of our own Caribbean authors release such a powerful book. I highly recommend this and all of Dr Fagan's books. Maureen Hamilton, CEO Avodah Productions & Ministries, Jamaica

I knew this is one book I had to share it with as many as I could. As an established author and publisher of several books I know good stuff when I see it. I endorse this book and commend Dr Juliette Fagan for all of her efforts in education the church and public at large. Dr Samuel McKenzie, UK

I ordered my copy after seeing the post on facebook. It is working wonders in our home; I am using it in my hair and telling all of my clients about this wonderful book. Beth Seemann, Colon Therapist, USA.

I am proud of the research work done by Dr J. Fagan to get this book published. It is a must read for everyone. M. Gibbons, Ja.

Book her for your next speaking engagement, healthy life styles seminar, church, school, business fair, chamber of commerce, conferences or organizational events.

Websites

Colon Therapy & Detox Centre:

www.healthysolutionsbiz.com

healthy_solutions@yahoo.com

Ministry & Bible School:

www.visionmiraclecog.info

visionmiraclecog@yahoo.com

ISBN 978-1-312-08314-1

9 781312 083141